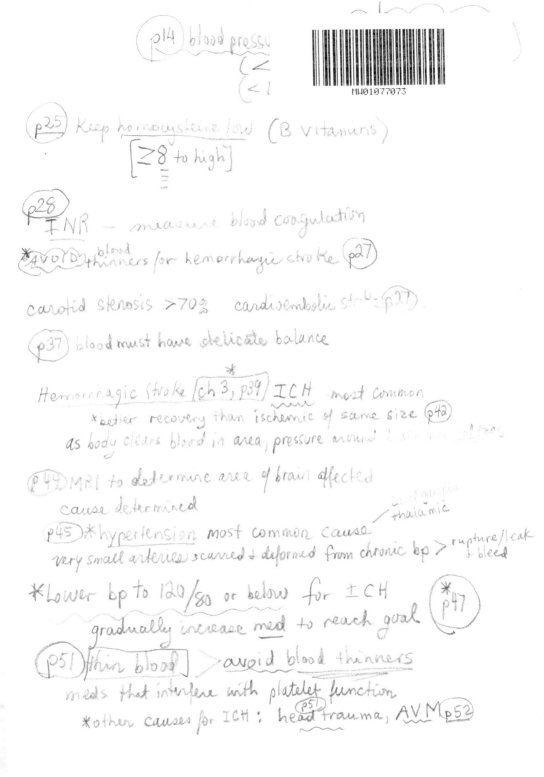

(p14) blood pressu

≤
< 1

(p25) Keep homocysteine low (B vitamins)

[≥ 8 to high]

(p28)
INR — measure blood coagulation

*AVOID blood thinners for hemorrhagic stroke (p27)

carotid stenosis > 70%   cardioembolic stroke (p27)

(p37) blood must have delicate balance

Hemorrhagic stroke [ch 3, p39] ICH   most common
        *better recovery than ischemic of same size (p42)
    as body clears blood in area, pressure around

(p44) MRI to determine area of brain affected
    cause determined
                                                        thalamic
    (p45) *hypertension most common cause
    very small arteries scarred & deformed from chronic bp > rupture/leak
                                                                 & bleed

*Lower bp to 120/80 or below for ICH   (*p47)
        gradually increase med to reach goal

(p51) thin blood > avoid blood thinners
    meds that interfere with platelet function
        *other causes for ICH : head trauma, AVM (p52)
                                        (p51)

STOP YOUR NEXT STROKE

Stroke prevention for those who have had a stroke
or stroke-like symptom

David Alway, M.D.

Board Certified Neurologist and Chairman of the
Stroke Clinical Effectiveness Team at
Alexandria Hospital, Virginia

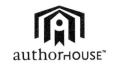

authorHOUSE™

1663 Liberty Drive, Suite 200
Bloomington, Indiana 47403
(800) 839-8640
www.AuthorHouse.com

First published by AuthorHouse 12/16/05

ISBN: 1-4208-5612-X (sc)

Printed in the United States of America
Bloomington, Indiana

This book is printed on acid-free paper.

DISCLAIMER

The information contained in this book is not intended as a substitute for the advice of a treating physician or other health care professional. Indeed, this book and the included Goal Chart are intended to be used with your physician to pursue a set of patient-specific stroke prevention goals.

Table of Contents

Introduction ix

Chapter 1: Strokes And Stroke Types 1

Chapter 2: Ischemic Strokes (And TIAs) 3

Chapter 3: Hemorrhagic Strokes 39

Chapter 4: Putting It All Together..............57

Appendix A – Warfarin Use 61

Appendix B – What To Do If You're Having A
Stroke...63

Stroke Prevention Goal Charts 67

Endnotes 75

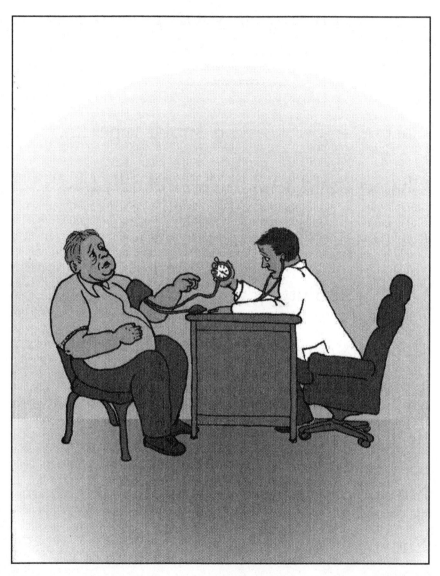

"Can you recommend any supplements for stroke prevention?"

INTRODUCTION

If you have suffered from a stroke or stroke-like episode, you are not alone. Roughly 700,000 new strokes occur each year and 4.4 million people are stroke survivors in the United States. If you include those who have suffered from temporary stroke-like episodes (transient ischemic attacks or TIAs), this will add 4.9 million, bringing the total number to 9.3 million survivors. Stroke is the number one cause of disability and the third-leading cause of death in the United States. More worrisome is the fact that once you have suffered from a stroke or stroke-like episode, your chances of having another stroke are dramatically increased. Between 25-40% of stroke patients and 25-30% of TIA patients will have a first stroke or a recurrent stroke within the next five years. Fortunately, numerous steps can be taken to significantly reduce your chances of having a stroke. This guide will provide you with the knowledge and tools necessary to develop your own personal plan for stroke prevention.

I am a neurologist with a special interest in stroke and its prevention. As part of my daily practice, I advise patients about aspects of their lives and health they can change to reduce their stroke risk. Despite my advice regarding the *most important* and *proven* ways to reduce stroke risk, I am continually surprised to discover my patients focusing on minor or unproven treatments for stroke prevention. One reason for this phenomenon is probably the extraneous and potentially contradictory information on stroke prevention provided by the mass media. Also, it is much easier to take a vitamin supplement, for example, than to work on difficult issues such as quitting smoking or losing weight. This book is an easy-to-read guide that will reorient stroke and TIA patients on stroke prevention *essentials*. You can use it to develop your own plan of prevention, based on your stroke type and risk factors. The prevention plan that results will be 'do-able,' that is, not overwhelming, but also will cover 99% of what can be done to prevent strokes.

The Goal Chart, which accompanies this book, is the key to its organization. The Goal Chart lists many goals, some of which it will be appropriate for you to follow and others which you should ignore. Which goals you select will depend on what type of stroke you have had and the probable cause. As you read through the book, you will learn which goals are appropriate for your situation and you will be asked to place an 'X' next to those goals on the chart. When you have finished the book, you can then use the Goal Chart as a reminder of your goals and to track your progress as you achieve them. To the right of the goals are blank spaces to record either 'yes' or 'no' regarding having achieved a goal, or to write the relevant value for that date. If you bring the chart along when you visit your doctor, it will also help him or her follow your progress and give appropriate advice or make medication changes.

In the first chapter of the book, some general information about strokes is presented and you will also learn about your stroke type. Depending on your stroke type, you will then either be referred to Chapter 2 (Ischemic Strokes) or Chapter 3 (Hemorrhagic Strokes). After reading the appropriate chapter for your stroke type, you should then read Chapter 4 (Putting It All Together).

CHAPTER 1: STROKES AND STROKE TYPES

The brain requires a steady supply of oxygen and glucose in order to function and remain alive. This is supplied by the continuous circulation of blood through arteries to all areas of your brain. The blood then exits the brain through large veins. Each area of the brain has a different function. For example, some regions of the brain can cause facial movement; others can cause movements of your arms or legs. Different brain areas are involved in the sensation of touch for your face, or torso, or extremities. Brain areas can be very specialized – controlling eye movements, speech perception, visual perception, coordination, and more.

In the event the blood supply to a portion of the brain is interrupted, symptoms will persist for the duration of the interruption. For example, if the blood supply to the areas of the brain involved in right-arm movement and language production is interrupted, then the person will experience weakness of the right arm and difficulty speaking. Let's suppose such an event does occur, with reestablishment of the blood supply after about 10 minutes. In this case, the person will experience weakness of the right arm and decreased ability to speak for 10 minutes – regaining these functions fully once the blood supply is reestablished. Medical doctors refer to this event as a *transient ischemic attack* (TIA). Ischemia refers to *starvation* of brain tissue for lack of adequate oxygen and glucose. Now in this same case, if the blood supply is *not* reestablished, the brain region, being starved of oxygen and glucose, will eventually die. This event is referred to as an *ischemic stroke.*

The other major type of stroke is called *hemorrhagic* stroke. This stroke-type is usually due to bleeding in or around the brain from one of its arteries. If the bleeding is deep within the substance of the brain, it is referred to as an *intracerebral hemorrhage* (ICH). If the bleeding is into the fluid that surrounds the brain (cerebrospinal fluid), it is referred to as a *subarachnoid hemorrhage* (SAH).

If you don't already know, you should learn which of these stroke types applies to you and then read the chapter in this book that deals with your stroke type. Read Chapter 2 if you suffered from an ischemic stroke or TIA. Read Chapter 3 if you suffered from an intracerebral hemorrhage or subarachnoid hemorrhage.

Chapter 2: Ischemic Strokes (And TIAs)

HOW ISCHEMIC STROKES AND TIAs OCCUR

Ischemic stroke is the most common type of stroke, accounting for about 85% of all strokes. The best thing about having had an ischemic stroke (or TIA) is that typically you can do many things to reduce your risk of having another one.

The most important question regarding ischemic stroke is: What caused the stroke? The answer is usually one of three:

(1) An already narrow (atherosclerotic) artery in the brain or neck closes completely (see Diagram 1).

(2) A blood clot breaks off from an (atherosclerotic) artery and travels downstream, finally blocking a smaller artery in the brain (see Diagram 2).

(3) A blood clot from the heart travels to an artery in the brain, blocking blood flow in that artery (see Diagram 3).

We will discuss rarer causes of ischemic stroke later in this chapter. Despite a thorough evaluation, in about 30% of cases, the cause of an ischemic stroke is not discovered.

ISCHEMIC STROKE PREVENTION

This chapter divides ischemic stroke prevention into three sections: (1) Preventing Clot Formation; (2) Preventing or Reversing Atherosclerosis; and (3) Special Causes and Treatments of Ischemic Stroke.

Preventing Clot Formation

Platelets are small flat blood cells that help blood to clot. It has been proven, through numerous scientific studies, that medications which interfere with the functioning of platelets (making them less 'sticky' and therefore less likely to clot) reduce your chances of having an ischemic stroke. Sometimes doctors will use another medication, Coumadin

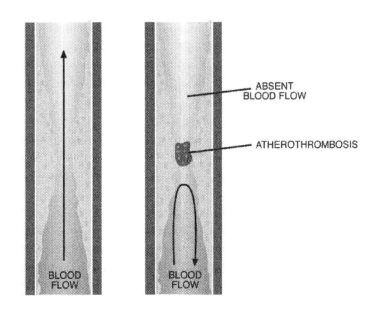

Diagram 1

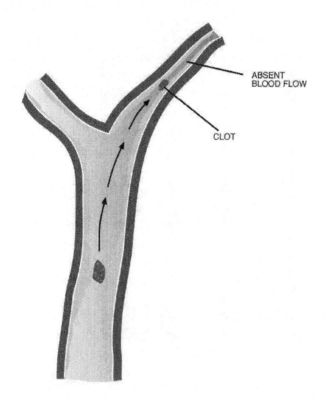

ABSENT
BLOOD FLOW

CLOT

Diagram 2

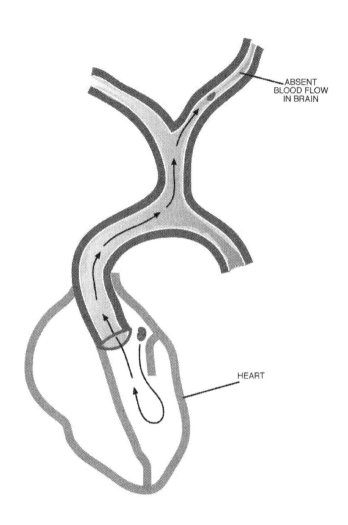

ABSENT
BLOOD FLOW
IN BRAIN

HEART

Diagram 3

(generic name warfarin), which does not affect platelets but also prevents clot formation. Any person who has suffered from an ischemic stroke should take either an antiplatelet medication or Coumadin daily. If you have had an ischemic stroke or TIA and are not taking Coumadin, place an 'X' next to the 'Antiplatelet' goal on your Ischemic Stroke Goal Chart. The most common clot-preventing medications used for stroke prevention are listed below:

Coumadin (warfarin) - This medication is usually taken at bedtime. The dose varies greatly and is adjusted according to periodic measures of your blood's clotting tendency (INR). Taking this medication can be complicated, so please read Appendix A for helpful ideas regarding its use.

Antiplatelet Medications:

Aspirin 81-325mg taken once a day. This antiplatelet medication is still considered very effective and is certainly the cheapest available. There is a trend towards using the lowest dose (81mg) to avoid stomach problems such as gastritis and ulcers.

Aggrenox (aspirin 25mg/dipyridamole 200mg) taken twice a day. Aggrenox is probably the best antiplatelet medication since it greatly reduces one's chances of having an ischemic stroke and is not usually associated with serious side effects.

<u>Plavix</u> (clopidogrel) 75mg taken once a day. Plavix is about as effective as aspirin for ischemic stroke prevention. It is a good choice for those who are aspirin intolerant.

<u>Ticlid</u> (ticlopidine) 250mg taken twice a day. Ticlid is probably more effective than aspirin in terms of stroke prevention, but is used by few neurologists due to rare but potentially serious side effects (Thrombotic Thrombocytopenic Purpura).

Preventing or Reversing Atherosclerosis

If you review the common causes of ischemic stroke, you will notice that the first two causes mentioned (see Diagrams 1 and 2), involve the process of atherosclerosis or 'hardening' of the arteries. You can think of atherosclerosis as a chronic inflammation or irritation of an artery, causing the walls of the artery to thicken over time. The inflammation and build-up are caused by cholesterol deposits and inflammatory cells. This inflammation can cause the artery to become completely blocked, in severe cases, or it can cause *blood clots* to form, which can then travel into the brain and cause a stroke.

Clearly if we could avoid the process of atherosclerosis we could dramatically reduce our chances of having an ischemic

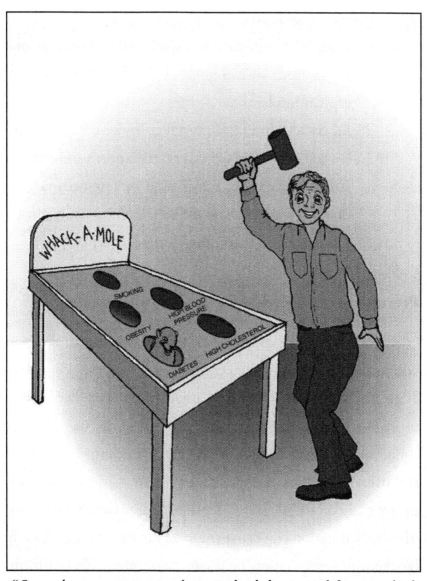

"Over the years, scientists have indeed discovered factors which worsen or improve atherosclerosis."

stroke. Over the years, scientists have indeed discovered factors which worsen or improve atherosclerosis. For example, smoking and elevated LDL cholesterol ('bad' cholesterol) appear to exacerbate atherosclerosis while weight loss and cholesterol-lowering medications appear to improve it. There is even evidence, in both cardiac and stroke literature, that atherosclerosis can be *reversed* - excellent news if you have suffered an ischemic stroke or TIA caused by atherosclerosis, since aggressively reversing the process may mean never having another stroke!

But how do you know if you suffer from atherosclerosis? Neurologists who treat stroke don't always have the answer to this question. In many cases, you may already have a diagnosis that indicates you have a problem with atherosclerosis. For example, if you suffer from coronary artery disease, then you have atherosclerotic disease. You are included in this group if you have suffered from angina, have had a heart attack, or have had heart bypass surgery or a cardiac stent. If you have peripheral vascular disease then you suffer from atherosclerosis. You are included in this group if you experience pain in the legs after sustained walking (claudication), have undergone bypass surgery in the legs, or are known to have poor arterial circulation in your legs. If you are known to have plaque (atherosclerotic build-up) in any of the blood vessels in or leading to your brain, then you suffer from atherosclerosis. If it is still unclear to you whether or not you suffer from this problem, you may need to speak with your doctor about it. In most cases, unless there is a clear alternate cause of your stroke or TIA, the cause is assumed to be atherosclerosis and you are advised to follow the advice below regarding preventing or reversing atherosclerosis.

Blood Sugar:

Your blood sugar (glucose level) should be monitored only if you have been diagnosed with diabetes (diabetes mellitus) or impaired glucose tolerance. If this describes you, please place an 'X' next to the 'Blood Sugar' goal on your chart. You should work closely with your primary care physician or diabetes specialist to keep your average glucose in the normal range. Sometimes your doctor will have you check your glucose level periodically using a glucometer. Sometimes your doctor will perform a blood test (hemoglobin A1c), which measures your average blood glucose level over the past three months. The more normal you can get your average glucose level, the less chance you will develop (and the greater your chances of reversing) atherosclerosis.

Blood Pressure:

Blood pressure is measured in millimeters of Mercury (mm Hg) and is divided into two numbers. The first number (systolic blood pressure) refers to the pressure of the blood in your arteries while your heart is pumping. The second number (diastolic blood pressure) refers to the pressure of your blood while your heart is relaxing between beats. If you suffer from atherosclerosis, lowering your blood pressure is one of the best methods of reducing your chances of having another stroke. Chronically elevated blood pressure damages the walls of arteries, accelerating the process of atherosclerosis.

But how much should your blood pressure be lowered? Interestingly, from the standpoint of atherosclerosis prevention, evidence suggests there is no lower limit! Again, from the standpoint of atherosclerosis development, the lower your blood pressure the better.[1] Estimates are that for each 5-6mm of mercury reduction in diastolic blood pressure, your stroke risk reduces by 35-40%.[2] Of course, if your blood pressure dips too low, you will develop other problems such as lightheadedness, fatigue, or actually passing out! The most informed recommendations come from the committee that studies hypertension: The Joint National Committee on the Prevention, Detection, Evaluation, and Treatment of High Blood Pressure.[3] According to the committee's recommendations, which take the latest information on stroke prevention into account, normal blood pressure is anything below 120 systolic and 80 diastolic. If your blood pressure is higher than 120/80, and you have suffered from a TIA or ischemic stroke, it should be brought down to these levels. Place an 'X' next to the 'Blood Pressure' goal on your Goal Chart.

To lower your blood pressure, you can begin by focusing on weight loss and a low salt diet, which may allow you to bring your blood pressure into the recommended range. If these measures are not effective within a few months, you should have your doctor prescribe medication to lower your blood pressure (see below). Since you may not be able to tolerate blood pressures below 120/80mm Hg (due to lightheadedness upon standing or generalized fatigue) your doctor's goal will be to lower your blood pressure just above the level at which you begin to experience these symptoms. It is possible that over time, as you become tolerant of lower blood pressures, you will eventually be able to tolerate pressures at the recommended levels.

The stroke literature suggests there might be a special benefit in being on *certain types* of blood pressure medications called thiazide diuretics and ACE-inhibitors.[4] [5] [6] For this reason, if you have even a hint of elevated blood pressure, you would probably benefit from being on a thiazide diuretic, an ACE-inhibitor, or a combination of the two. Ask your doctor which medication is appropriate for your circumstance.

*chlorthalidone
(hydrochlorothiazide)*

120s
130s
140s

Smoking:

Smoking is clearly a dangerous habit if continued for many years due to increased risk of lung cancer, emphysema, and heart attacks. Smoking is also a powerful contributor to stroke risk. One group of scientists [7] pooled the data from multiple studies examining the relationship between ischemic stroke risk and smoking. They found that a person's chances of suffering an ischemic stroke almost doubles (a relative risk of 1.9) if that person smokes. Also, there appears to be a clear dose-response relationship. In other words, the more a person smokes, the higher the stroke risk. This increased risk is probably due to multiple mechanisms, including accelerated atherosclerosis [8] and an increased tendency for blood to clot in smokers.

Because smoking is such a large contributor to atherosclerosis, it is a 'no-brainer' that anyone who has had a stroke or TIA should stop. If you smoke, you should place an 'X' next to the goal of 'No Smoking' on your Goal Chart. Many people, of course, find quitting to be extremely difficult. The pleasure from the nicotine rush, combined with the significant pain of an extended withdrawal, is difficult for many to overcome. If you've had a stroke or TIA, then motivation should not be a problem for you. If you need more motivation, then consider the good news: If you quit smoking, your risk returns to that of a non-smoker after only 5 years.[9] In other words, if you can stop smoking for 5 years, you have essentially eliminated this risk factor from your life.

Quitting smoking, I think, should be approached in the same way that you pursue any important goal in life. You should work on a plan to quit smoking in the same manner you would plan to develop your career, lose weight, buy a house, or learn a new language. You need a long-term plan for quitting. Study the problem; study your own motivations, the situations that make you more likely to smoke, and your feelings regarding quitting. Set aside time to plan how you can quit. You should consider using over-the-counter medications (nicotine patch, nicotine gum), getting medications (Zyban) from your doctor, attending classes, or going to specialized clinics for smoking cessation. Treat smoking cessation as the life-altering accomplishment that it is and something worth the effort.

Alcohol Intake:

When it comes to ischemic stroke or TIAs, alcohol is not necessarily bad. In fact, it may be helpful. It all depends on the 'dose.' Various studies [10] [11] [12] [13] lend support to the concept that a small amount of daily alcohol can act as a stroke *preventative,* while larger amounts of alcohol can make stroke more likely. Certainly, then, if you already drink alcohol, the best approach is to keep your intake within the recommended limit. The amount varies according to your gender. Because the stomach of men metabolizes alcohol more easily, they can, on average, tolerate larger amounts:

(1) Women: no more than 1 alcoholic drink* per day.
(2) Men: no more than two alchoholic drinks* per day.

*A drink is defined as 12 ounces of beer or wine cooler, 5 ounces of wine, or 1.5 ounces of 80-proof distilled spirits.

Since most doctors have a hard time *recommending* alcohol intake, they don't generally tell you to start drinking if you don't already drink (perhaps for fear that this will inadvertently lead to alcoholism). But, if you have been avoiding alcohol for any perceived health reason, you can certainly use the above evidence to support drinking lightly! You should check with you doctor, though, to make sure alcohol will not interfere with any of your medications. If appropriate, place an 'X' next to the 'Alcohol' goal on your Goal Chart and circle the appropriate per-day drink limit.

Exercise:

Exercise can reduce your stroke risk, independent of its effect on weight loss. One important study found that, in men, those who performed moderate exercise had a significantly lower stroke risk compared to those who did almost no exercise.[14] A later study found that the more you exercise (no matter your ethnicity or gender), the more benefit in terms of stroke risk reduction.[15]

Scientists still disagree on the 'right' amount of exercise one should do. Part of the problem is that 'amount' of exercise is difficult to measure and the significance of different ways of exercising is difficult to tease out. Is walking for an hour as beneficial as jogging for 15 minutes? Because of these difficulties, scientists at the National Institutes of Health convened a panel to discuss general recommendations regarding the appropriate amount of exercise (NIH Consensus Development Panel on Physical Activity and Cardiovascular health.) [16] To reduce one's chances of cardiovascular disease (including stroke and heart attacks), they recommend 30 minutes a day of moderately intense physical activity on most, and preferably all, days of the week. Moderately intense physical activity includes activities such as brisk walking, cycling, swimming, home repair, or yard work. Such activities are aerobic exercise in that they tend to involve sustained activity of multiple muscle groups and lead to a substantial increase in your heart and respiratory rates.

Abiding by the NIH Consensus recommendations is quite difficult for the majority of busy people or for those who are significantly overweight. Because of this, if you currently *rarely* or *never* exercise, I recommend that you perform some form of cardiovascular exercise at least 30 minutes a day, three times a week. This represents your 'bare minimum' goal and is a good starting point. If you have significant weakness or poor balance due to a prior stroke, then you should work with your physical therapist to develop exercises that will allow you to achieve increased heart and respiratory rates. Place an 'X' next to the 'Aerobic Exercise' goal on your Goal Chart. Once this goal (and your other chart goals) has been achieved, you can then revisit the issue and consider more frequent or more intense exercise goals that will provide even more benefit from the standpoint of stroke prevention.

Weight:

Obesity is clearly a strong contributor to ischemic stroke risk. A large part of this contribution stems from its tendency to exacerbate other conditions we've already discussed, such as hypertension, diabetes, and cholesterol profile.[17] [18] Obesity can be measured in different ways but it appears that measures of central obesity (or abdominal obesity) are greater predictors of cardiovascular disease than other measures (such as Body Mass Index).[19] One recent study[20] finds that Waist-to-Hip Ratio is a potent risk factor for ischemic stroke. This risk remains even when the effects of other risk factors (hypertension, diabetes, cholesterol profiles) are statistically eliminated. Even when the effects of another measure of obesity (Body Mass Index) are eliminated, the adverse effect of central obesity remains. So Waist-to-Hip Ratio appears to be the best measure of obesity for the purposes of stroke prevention. Please place an 'X' next to the 'Waist-to-Hip Ratio' goal on your Goal Chart.

How is Waist-to-Hip Ratio (WHR) measured and what is an appropriate goal? Using a flexible tape measure, record your waist measurement at the level of your umbilicus (belly-button). The measurement can be done in inches or centimeters. Your hip is measured at the level where you can feel your greater trochanter (the top of your upper leg bone) or the level of greatest distance around your hips and buttocks (see Diagram 4). Divide the waist number by the hip number to get the ratio. Since men, on average, have smaller hips, their goal ratio is higher. For men the goal WHR is less than 0.93 and for women it is less than 0.86. On the chart, circle the appropriate goal for you and record your current WHR in the blank to the right.

Special Notes. If you are significantly overweight, your chances of having obstructive sleep apnea or glucose intolerance are markedly increased. Please read the following two sections to see if they apply to you:

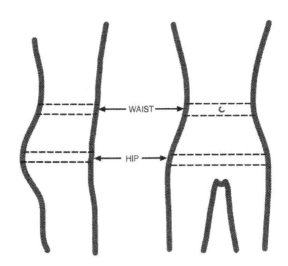

Diagram 4

Obstructive Sleep Apnea (OSA) – Obstructive sleep apnea is a condition of disrupted breathing while a person is asleep caused by collapse of the back of the throat. It can rob an individual of a good night's sleep, without that person being aware of the problem. If you are consistently sleepy, and are significantly overweight, there is a chance that you have obstructive sleep apnea. Many people who have this condition snore loudly while they are asleep and some are observed by others to have significant pauses in their breathing while asleep. OSA contributes to a worse quality of life (since it makes people feel chronically tired). It can also significantly increase your risk of a stroke or cardiac arrhythmia. As the experts summarize, OSA "affects almost every system in the body, resulting in an increased incidence of hypertension, cardiovascular disease, stroke, pulmonary hypertension, cardiac arrhythmias, and altered immune function."[21] If you are significantly overweight and feel chronically sleepy, you should ask your doctor about being tested for obstructive sleep apnea. If you are diagnosed with it, place an 'X' next to the 'Obstructive Sleep Apnea' goal on your chart. Your doctor will need to consider options such as placing you on a night-time breathing aid (CPAP or BiPAP), weight loss, or, occasionally, surgical intervention.

Impaired Glucose Tolerance – Impaired glucose tolerance refers to the inability of your body to keep your glucose (blood sugar) levels within a normal range. You can look at it as a mild form of diabetes and certainly it can be a precursor to the development of diabetes. If you are significantly overweight and you have had an ischemic stroke or TIA before the age of 45, you should undergo a glucose tolerance test to check for this problem. If you are diagnosed with this problem, place an 'X' next to the 'Impaired Glucose Tolerance' goal on your chart. Treatments by your doctor might include weight counseling, a special diet, or oral medications to help lower your glucose.

Cholesterol and Triglycerides:

It is probably no news to you that cholesterol and triglycerides are highly linked to stroke and heart attack risk.[22] [23] You probably also know that there are different categories of cholesterol, such as Low-Density Lipoprotein (LDL-C) and High-Density Lipoprotein (HDL-C). When it comes to ischemic stroke prevention, the biggest emphasis is on lowering your LDL cholesterol. I follow the recommendations of The American Heart Association, which advocates lowering LDL-C below 100mg/dL for those who have suffered from a stroke or heart attack. While there is the possibility that LDL values even *lower* than 100mg/dL would be of benefit, there is not yet much evidence to support this goal.

Your level of triglycerides and HDL should also be examined. If triglycerides (TG) are greater than 150mg/dL or HDL-C less than 40mg/dL, you should pursue weight loss and exercise to try to lower them. If these are not effective, you should take certain medications (statins, fibrates, or niacin) to lower them. If your TG level is greater than 200, it is recommended you pursue exercise, weight loss, *and* treat with one of the medications mentioned above (since it is unlikely you will be able to sufficiently lower the values through weight loss and exercise alone). Please place an 'X' next to LDL, TG, and HDL on your Goal Chart.

Statin Medications:

While no one wants to take medications unnecessarily, certain medications might prevent you from having a stroke, even if you don't have the condition they were originally intended to treat. The best examples of these are the statin drugs (HMG-CoA reductase inhibitors such as prava*statin*, lova*statin*, simva*statin*). While these medications are effective in improving a person's cholesterol profile, they seem also to have an anti-inflammatory effect, which reverses or prevents atherosclerosis, even in people who already have a good cholesterol profile.[24] Based on this information, any patient with atherosclerosis as the cause of his or her stroke should strongly consider taking a statin medication. Please place an 'X' next to 'Statin' on your Goal Chart.

Homocysteine:

Homocysteine is an amino acid that circulates in the blood. Amino acids are the building blocks of proteins in your body, so it is essential to have a certain amount of homocysteine in your body. Unfortunately, an excess of homocysteine leads to increased inflammation of arterial walls (atherosclerosis). Children can be born with a genetic defect that causes dramatic rises in homocysteine levels (Homocystinuria). The effect of super-elevated homocysteine levels is so dramatic that these children have strokes at very young ages.

Everyone is potentially susceptible to the effects of even a moderate increase in blood homocysteine levels. Experts believe that a large number of people have slight genetic defects that lead to moderate increases in homocysteine levels. Also, people who have kidney disease, especially those on dialysis, have a poor ability to excrete homocysteine, leading to elevated blood levels.

Homocysteine can be reduced by fostering its rapid metabolism (breakdown) and reducing its formation. These processes are encouraged by taking vitamins B6, B12, and folic acid. While it has been proven that taking these vitamins can reduce homocysteine levels, *it has yet to be proven that this treatment definitely reduces the chances of having a stroke.*[25] Still, since the treatment is so simple and safe, with the potential for benefit, I recommend monitoring and treating elevated homocysteine levels. Place an 'X' next to the 'Homocysteine' goal on your Goal Chart.

If your homocysteine level is equal to or greater than 8 microM/L you can initially start by taking 25mg of vitamin B6, 1mg of vitamin B12, and 2.5mg of folic acid daily. These vitamins can be bought separately or you can get a prescription for Foltx, a single pill that includes all three vitamins in these doses. If your homocysteine levels do not go down adequately after taking these vitamins for a month, you should double the dose of each. If you are still not in the goal range, after doubling your vitamin doses, you should still remain on the vitamins to keep your homocysteine levels as low as possible.

SPECIAL CAUSES AND TREATMENTS OF ISCHEMIC STROKE:

If you have any of the conditions mentioned in the following section, please read the special advice that follows:

Cardioembolic Source:

If your doctor has determined that your stroke (or TIA) was due to a blood clot that originated in your heart, you are a special case. Generally, in such a case, you will be placed on a blood thinner called warfarin (brand name: Coumadin). One reason to suspect that the heart is the culprit is the discovery of an abnormal heart rhythm (such as atrial fibrillation or sick sinus syndrome). When the heart does not beat correctly, it causes blood to pool within its chambers. Blood that pools has a greater tendency to clot. Once formed, a clot may then be ejected out of the heart, through the arteries that lead to the brain, causing an ischemic stroke or TIA. Other reasons the heart can form clots include: artificial (metallic or porcine) heart valves, a recent heart attack (myocardial infarction) or a heart that beats very weakly (very low ejection fraction).

Your doctor may not put you on warfarin if he or she feels it is too risky in your case. For example, it might be unsafe to put you on warfarin if you have had a hemorrhagic stroke in the past, tend to be unsteady and are at risk of falling, or have had excessive bleeding in another part of your body. If you are not on warfarin, you should at least take an antiplatelet medication.

If you have suffered a stroke or TIA due to a cardioembolic source and are taking warfarin, please read Appendix A

27

regarding warfarin use and the measurement of blood coagulation (INR). Place an 'X' next to the 'Monitor INR'; goal on your Goal Chart and ask your physician what INR range he or she is trying to achieve (usually 2.0-3.0). You should write that range in the blank provided on the chart. In addition, if you smoke, you should put an 'X' next to the 'No Smoking' goal on your chart and then read the section in this chapter regarding smoking. In your case, smoking is harmful because it makes it more likely that your heart will form blood clots and cause a stroke. Finally, you should contact your doctor to find out if you have any condition (coronary artery disease, peripheral vascular disease, etc.) that would warrant aggressively treating atherosclerosis. If you have such a condition you should be sure to follow all of the advice under the 'Preventing or Reversing Atherosclerosis' section of this chapter.

Carotid Stenosis:

The carotid arteries are large blood vessels in the neck that lead to the brain (see Diagram 5). As shown, the common carotid artery splits into an external and an internal portion. Unfortunately, the region where the artery splits (the carotid bulb) is typically where atherosclerosis (inflammation and thickening of the vessel wall) develops. This atherosclerosis can lead to a stroke by closing off the entire artery, stopping all blood flow through it and to the brain (Diagram 6). Alternatively, a portion of the atherosclerotic wall can break open and cause the blood in that region to clot. This clot can then break off and travel up the internal carotid artery into the brain, leading to an ischemic stroke (Diagram 7).

If you have been diagnosed with plaque in your carotid arteries, then you definitely have atherosclerosis and need to follow the advice in the section 'Preventing or Reversing Atherosclerosis.' In addition, though, if the degree of narrowing (stenosis) in your carotid artery is severe enough, you may benefit by having the artery widened again (by various means). Just how much narrowing should exist in order to have the problem corrected is still a matter of controversy and seems to depend on a lot of other factors including the skill of the physicians performing the procedure and your overall health. In addition, the artery that is on the same side of your brain as the stroke (symptomatic carotid stenosis) is more important to correct than narrowing on the other side (asymptomatic carotid stenosis). The following advice is considered by most to be non-controversial:

o If you have 70-99% carotid stenosis on the same side of the brain as your stroke, you will likely benefit from a procedure to eliminate the stenosis, assuming your overall health is reasonably good.

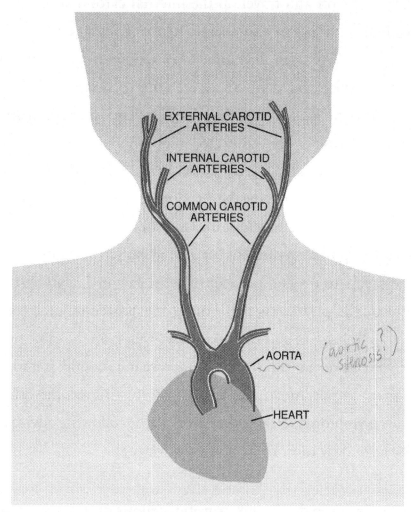

Diagram 5

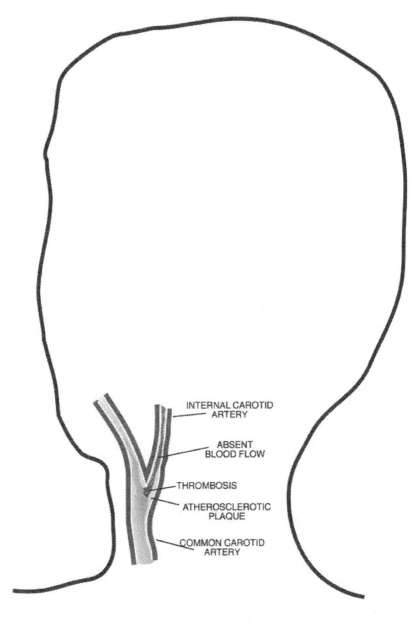

INTERNAL CAROTID
ARTERY

ABSENT
BLOOD FLOW

THROMBOSIS

ATHEROSCLEROTIC
PLAQUE

COMMON CAROTID
ARTERY

Diagram 6

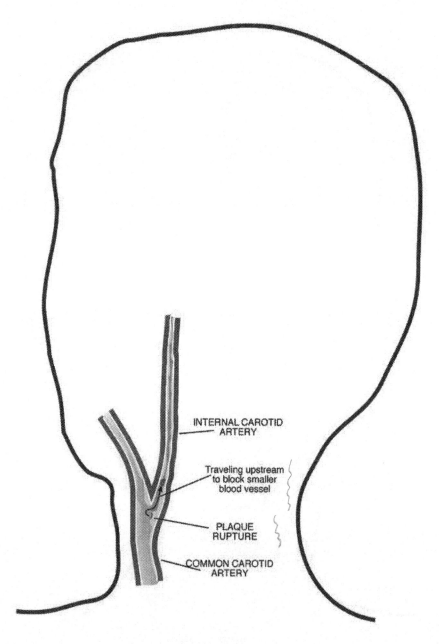

INTERNAL CAROTID
ARTERY

Traveling upstream
to block smaller
blood vessel

PLAQUE
RUPTURE

COMMON CAROTID
ARTERY

Diagram 7

o If you are older than 85 years, your chances of suffering from a stroke while undergoing a corrective procedure is high (12-15%) and you should consider this option with your physician very carefully, weighing the risks and benefits.

If you have decided, with your doctor, that you will have a procedure to correct the problem, you must then decide which procedure is right for you. One choice is surgical removal of the atherosclerotic plaque, referred to as *carotid endarterectomy* (CEA). This is a time-honored procedure for which there is a lot of data and experience. Sometimes, though, because of your own special anatomy, the surgery is difficult to accomplish and you must be considered for another procedure called *carotid stenting*. In this procedure there is no overt surgery. Instead, a wire is threaded into an artery in your leg up to the internal carotid artery. Then an expandable tube of mesh (stent) is enlarged until it widens the artery at that location. The tube is left in place, where it eventually is covered by the artery's normal cells (endothelial cells).

Some patients would be appropriate for either procedure and current data suggests both procedures are likely to be equally effective. If this is your case, the particular experience of the physicians involved will be a critical issue. You will likely benefit from having the procedure done in a 'large volume' center, where the experience of the physicians is very high.

If you have at least a 50% stenosis in one or both or your internal carotid arteries, you should undergo carotid imaging (either carotid ultrasound [also called duplex] scanning or a magnetic resonance angiogram of the carotids) at least every 6 months. Having repeat evaluations of your carotid arteries can be particularly rewarding if you follow the advice in the section 'Preventing or Reversing Atherosclerosis,' since you might be pleasantly surprised to see a reduction in the degree of stenosis. If the degree of stenosis falls below 50%, you can probably wait a year before undergoing re-imaging of the carotids. If you undergo surgery or stenting to correct your carotid stenosis, your surgeon or interventional radiologist will determine at what intervals your carotid arteries should be evaluated. In any case, please place an 'X' next to the 'Carotid Imaging' goal if you have more than 50% stenosis in either internal carotid artery or if you have undergone a corrective procedure.

Arterial Dissection:

Arterial dissection is simply a tear in the wall of an artery (see Diagram 8). It most commonly affects the aorta (the largest artery in the body, located in your chest and abdomen), carotid arteries, and vertebral arteries (arteries in the back of

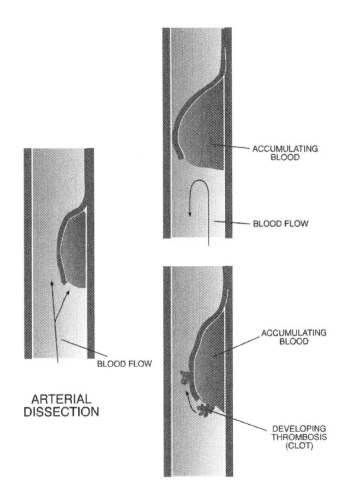

ACCUMULATING
BLOOD

BLOOD FLOW

ACCUMULATING
BLOOD

DEVELOPING
THROMBOSIS
(CLOT)

BLOOD FLOW

ARTERIAL
DISSECTION

Diagram 8

the neck) and often leads to pain in the location of the tear. While common causes of vertebral dissection include trauma and atherosclerosis, often no cause is discovered. A person will be more susceptible to an arterial dissection if he or she has a disease that leads to weakening in the structure of the artery such as Marfan syndrome, fibromuscular dysplasia, or Ehlers-Danlos syndrome.

Arterial dissections can cause a stroke in at least two ways. First, if the wall of the artery is expanded with blood, it can occlude (close) the main flow of blood, leading to an ischemic stroke. Second, because clotting can occur within the arterial wall and at the edges of the arterial tear, small clots of blood can travel upstream into the brain and cause an ischemic stroke. If you have been diagnosed with an arterial dissection, then you may have been placed on Coumadin (warfarin) to thin your blood. If this is the case, you should read Appendix A regarding warfarin use and coagulation (INR) monitoring. In addition, place an 'X' next to the 'Monitor INR' goal on your goal chart. Most stroke neurologists will continue anticoagulation medications until evidence of your dissection has resolved or at least until the blood vessel has become very stable (usually in 3-6 months). Since an arterial dissection is not necessarily due to atherosclerosis, you should ask your doctor if you suffer from atherosclerosis to see if you should follow the advice in the section 'Preventing or Reversing Atherosclerosis.' If you have a disease that makes you prone to arterial dissections, you should avoid any form of trauma to your head or neck – including avoiding chiropractic manipulation of your head and neck.

Hypercoagulable State:

Blood must maintain a delicate balance. While it needs to flow very easily under most circumstances; if the body is bleeding (for example, when you cut yourself) it also needs to *stop* flowing – or clot. Some people have blood that is out of balance and tends to clot when it shouldn't. There are many conditions that might cause blood to clot too easily. These include: cancer, Lupus, connective tissue diseases, deficiencies and excesses in clotting factors; and more common factors such as smoking or taking estrogen-containing birth control pills. If you've had an ischemic stroke or TIA due to one of these conditions, your doctor will likely place you on a blood thinning agent such as warfarin. If this is the case, you should become familiar with Appendix A regarding warfarin use and the coagulation test called INR and place an 'X' next to the 'Monitor INR' goal on your Goal Chart. You should also stop smoking (put an 'X' next to this goal on the Goal Chart) and stay off estrogen-containing birth control pills. You do not necessarily have a problem with atherosclerosis and therefore should speak with your doctor about whether you should follow the advice offered in the section 'Preventing or Reversing Atherosclerosis.' If you are a woman on estrogen-containing hormone-replacement therapy, you should probably stop this therapy, but should discuss this decision with your doctor first.

Rare Ischemic Stroke Causes:

There are many rarer causes of ischemic strokes that, if present in your case, will require the expertise of your doctor to discuss and treat. Examples of such conditions include: patent foramen ovale, vasculitis, mitochondria disease (MELAS), cocaine-induced vasospasm, systemic lupus erythematosis, sickle cell disease, Moyamoya disease, sepsis, endocarditis, neurosyphilis, systemic hypotension, neurofibromatosis, venous thrombosis, and polycythemia. Whether migraine headaches can cause ischemic strokes is still an unsettled question.

Turn now to Chapter 4 – Putting It All Together.

CHAPTER 3:
HEMORRHAGIC STROKES

As with ischemic strokes, hemorrhagic strokes come in many varieties and have different causes. Depending on what part of the brain is involved, and how large the hemorrhage is, one's disability can range from no disability at all to a very severe impairment even to the point of death. Hemorrhagic strokes are divided into the following types:

- Intracranial hemorrhage (ICH), which is bleeding into the substance of the brain. ICHs represent about 10% of all strokes (see Diagram 9).
- Subarachnoid hemorrhage (SAH), which is bleeding into the fluid that surrounds the brain (see Diagram 10). SAHs make up roughly 5% of all strokes.

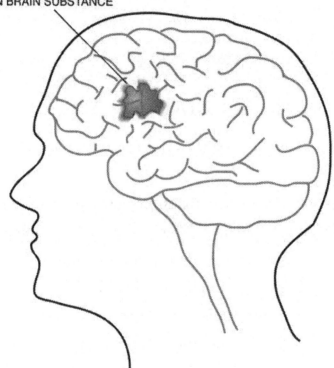

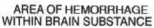

AREA OF HEMORRHAGE
WITHIN BRAIN SUBSTANCE

INTRACEREBRAL
HEMORRHAGE

Diagram 9

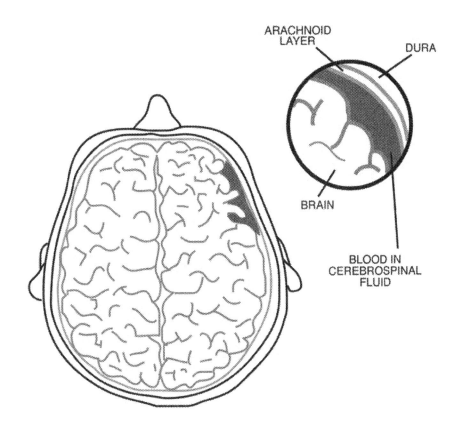

ARACHNOID LAYER

DURA

BRAIN

BLOOD IN CEREBROSPINAL FLUID

SUBARACHNOID HEMORRHAGE

Diagram 10

We will discuss the causes of hemorrhages later in this chapter when we discuss treatments.

In general, if an intracerebral hemorrhage and an ischemic stroke are of equal size, one tends to recover better from the hemorrhagic stroke. This is because some of the brain dysfunction from a hemorrhage occurs simply due to the pressure of blood on the surrounding brain. As the blood is cleared from the body over time, or through surgery, the pressure of the surrounding brain returns to normal and often there is then some return of normal function in these brain regions.

SAHs almost always occur due to the rupture of an aneurysm (an out pouching of a blood vessel – see Diagram 11). Compared to an ICH, the effects of SAHs are more complicated. Initially, there is the immediate effect of blood in the cerebrospinal fluid that surrounds the brain. The blood causes a severe headache and, if it interrupts the flow of the cerebrospinal fluid, can lead to markedly elevated pressure in the brain and even unconsciousness. Over the course of a few days this blood can also irritate the arteries that run through it. This arterial irritation can lead to spasm (small areas of narrowing) of the arteries, which can then cause an ischemic stroke.

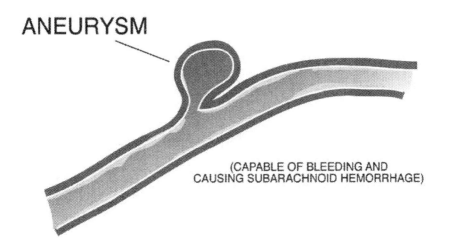

ANEURYSM

(CAPABLE OF BLEEDING AND
CAUSING SUBARACHNOID HEMORRHAGE)

Diagram 11

EVALUATING A HEMORRHAGIC STROKE: BRAIN IMAGING

In general, while a head computed tomography scan (head CT) is an excellent means of diagnosing a hemorrhagic stroke, it is not as good at identifying the potential causes of these strokes. Probably every hemorrhagic stroke patient deserves at least one brain magnetic resonance imaging (brain MRI). These scans are superior for identifying an underlying problem, such as a blood vessel malformation or tumor, which may have led to the hemorrhage. A brain MRA (magnetic resonance angiogram) is also useful to look at the blood vessels of the brain, as it may detect an aneurysm or other blood vessel anomaly. The gold standard, from the standpoint of evaluating the blood vessels of the brain, is a cerebral angiogram. This imaging study involves the threading of a wire catheter through a person's leg, up to the arteries that supply the brain. The catheter then releases a dye into the arteries, allowing very detailed x-ray pictures to be taken of the neck and brain arteries. Because there is always some risk involved with performing a cerebral angiogram, it should be undertaken only in special circumstances when a blood vessel abnormality is highly suspected.

If you have suffered from an intracranial hemorrhage, and your original brain MRI did not reveal an underlying cause of the bleed, you should have the MRI repeated in 3-4 months – since with clearing of the blood over time, a cause may indeed be detected. Place an 'X' next to the goal of 'Repeat Brain Imaging' on your Goal Chart.

CAUSES OF HEMORRHAGIC STROKE AND IMPLICATIONS FOR PREVENTION

Hypertension:

Hypertension is the most common cause of intracerebral hemorrhages. Typically, it can be assumed to be the cause of an ICH if a person has a known history of high blood pressure and the hemorrhage occurs in a typical *hypertensive location*. (Many brain locations are considered typical for hypertensive bleeds and they have names such as pons, thalamus, basal ganglia, or cerebellum). Scientists believe that with chronic exposure to elevated blood pressure, very small arteries (penetrating arteries) become scarred and deformed (lipohyalinosis). These arteries then develop defects in their walls (Charcot-Bouchard aneurysms) that can rupture and bleed.

High blood pressure is also a risk factor for subarachnoid hemorrhages,[26] [27] [28] [29] probably for two reasons. First, aneurysms are more likely to enlarge over time due to constant high internal pressure. Second, episodes of particularly high

45

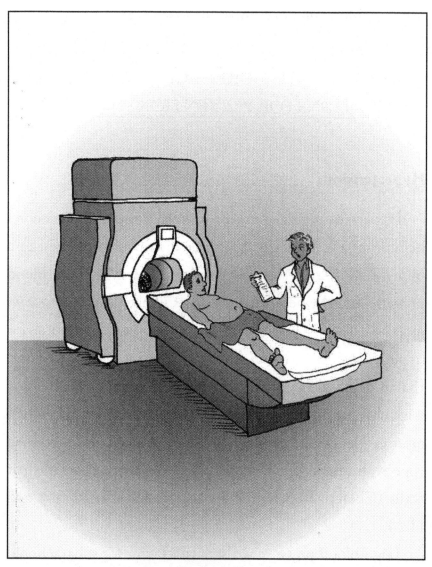

"You again!"

blood pressure, such as might occur if someone is upset or straining on the toilet with a bowel movement, will make aneurysms more likely to burst in that moment.

Prevention: If you have suffered from an ICH or SAH, your goal should be to lower your blood pressure to 120/80mm Hg or below.   Place an 'X' next to this goal on your Goal Chart in the hemorrhagic stroke section. You may initially start to reduce your blood pressure by avoiding salt in your diet and by losing weight. If these measures are not effective within a few months, you should be placed on an antihypertensive medication by your physician, gradually increasing the dose as necessary to reach this goal.

Alcohol:

Unlike the case of ischemic stroke, in which a small amount of alcohol is felt to be helpful, it seems the more alcohol you use, the higher your risk of a hemorrhagic stroke.[30] [31] [32] Alcoholics are at even higher risk, since excessive alcohol abuse can damage the liver to such a degree that it can no longer produce the clotting factors needed to clot blood. Any degree of alcohol ingestion, though, appears to increase the risk of hemorrhagic strokes.

Prevention: If you have suffered from a hemorrhagic stroke, you should probably avoid alcohol completely. Place an 'X' next to the 'Alcohol' goal on the Hemorrhagic Stroke Goal Chart.

Smoking:

There appears to be a direct relationship between the amount a person smokes and his or her risk of a subarachnoid hemorrhage or an intracerebral hemorrhage.[33] [34] However, one study found smoking to be a risk factor for intracerebral hemorrhage only in cases where hypertension was also present.[35]

Prevention: Despite the caveat above, clearly smoking is a risk factor for hemorrhagic strokes. You should place an 'X' next to the 'No Smoking' goal on your Goal Chart. Many people, of course, find quitting to be extremely difficult. The pleasure from the nicotine rush, combined with the significant pain of an extended withdrawal, is difficult for many to overcome. If you've had a hemorrhagic stroke, then motivation should not be a problem for you. If you need more motivation, then consider the good news: If you quit smoking, your stroke risk returns to that of a non-smoker after only 5 years [36]. In other words, if you can stop smoking for 5 years you have essentially eliminated this risk factor from you life.

Quitting smoking, I think, should be approached in the same way that you pursue any important goal in life. You should work on a plan to quit smoking in the same manner you would plan to develop your career, lose weight, buy a house, or learn a new language. You need a long-term plan for quitting. Study the problem; study your own motivations, the situations that make you more likely to smoke and your feelings regarding quitting. Set aside time to plan how you can quit. You should consider using over-the-counter medications (nicotine patch, nicotine gum), getting medications (Zyban) from your doctor, attending classes, or going to specialized clinics for smoking cessation. Treat smoking cessation as the life-altering accomplishment that it is and something worth the effort.

Cocaine and stimulants:

Cocaine, especially when injected or inhaled, can lead to sudden increases in blood pressure that can make an intracerebral hemorrhage or subarachnoid hemorrhage more likely to occur. Other stimulants, used as appetite suppressants, alerting medications, or decongestants, will also increase your risk of hemorrhagic stroke and should be avoided.

Prevention: Avoid illicit, prescription, or over-the-counter stimulants. Place an 'X' next to 'No Stimulants' on the Goal Chart. Please review the following list of common stimulant/ blood pressure elevating medications to avoid:

o Cocaine
o Amphetamine/dextroamphetamine (Brand names: Adderall, Dexadrine)
o Pemoline (Brand name: Cylert)
o Methylphenidate (Brand names: Metadate ER, Ritalin, Concerta)
o Appetite suppressants
o Pseudoephedrine
o Phenylpropanolamine

Bleeding Disorders:

Some people have blood that does not clot well. Often this is because they are taking a medication (such as wafarin [Coumadin]) that directly interferes in the clotting process. They may also be taking an antiplatelet medication, such as aspirin, Plavix, or Aggrenox, which causes an increased risk of bleeding. Some times their blood lacks the proper proteins involved in the clotting mechanism due to liver disease, or inherited conditions such as hemophilia, or Von Willebrand's disease.

Prevention: If the problem is related to taking blood thinners – you will generally want to avoid these medications. Place an 'X' next to 'No Blood Thinners' on your goal chart. If you must be on warfarin, please see Appendix A on 'Warfarin use' and learn about the coagulation measure called INR. You should also place an 'X' next to the 'Monitor INR' goal on your Goal Chart and write in the provided blank the INR goal your doctor wants to achieve. Generally, one would also want to avoid medications often used to treat ischemic stroke such as aspirin, ibuprofen, Aggrenox, Plavix, Ticlid, or any other medication which interferes with platelet function. There are special circumstances, though, in which your doctor may want you to be on one of these medications despite the increased risk of hemorrhage. Special bleeding disorders (such as hemophilia or Von Willebrand's disease) will require the expertise of your physician to manage.

Head Trauma:

Head trauma is a very common cause of both intracranial and subarachnoid hemorrhages. Usually the head trauma is very significant, such as may occur in a car accident or after a fall from a large height. On the other hand, in someone who has a bleeding disorder, the head trauma will not need to be as severe to produce the same result. Small bleeds near the surface of the brain, due to head trauma, are referred to as *contusions*.

<u>Prevention</u>: Clearly avoiding any form of head trauma is the key to prevention. This may also mean that if you have a history of falling easily, and have a bleeding disorder, or are on a blood thinner, you may need to walk with a cane, a walker, or even use a wheelchair to avoid falls. Sometimes your doctor will want to take you off warfarin (Coumadin) if you have a history of many falls.

Vascular Causes:

Abnormal blood vessels can lead to intracerebral hemorrhages or subarachnoid hemorrhages. Subarachnoid hemorrhages are almost always due to aneurysms, which are regions of arteries that balloon out (see Diagram 11) and can eventually burst. Arteries and veins can also grow together abnormally, forming a complex tangle of vessels called an arteriovenous malformation or AVM (see Diagram 12). This tangle of vessels bleeds much more easily than normal blood vessels. These malformations should be sought after more carefully if the location of a person's hemorrhage is not typical for hypertension, or if that person is not known to have hypertension. Usually a person will undergo special brain imaging (a brain magnetic resonance image [MRI] and a

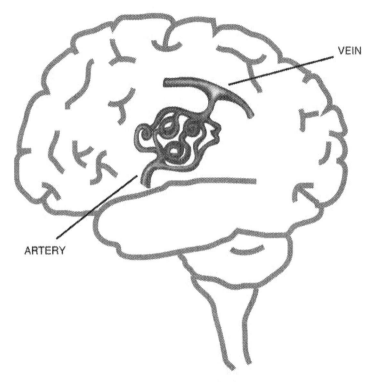

VEIN

ARTERY

ARTERIOVENOUS MALFORMATION

Diagram 12

magnetic resonance angiogram [MRA]) to look for evidence of these vascular problems. If no such cause is found, the MRI/MRA can be repeated in 3-4 months, when the blood has been cleared away, to look again for a vascular problem. Place an 'X' next to the goal of 'Repeat Brain Imaging' on your Goal Chart.

Prevention: The key to treatment is discovery of the vascular abnormality, as pointed out above, with good brain imaging. If a person is discovered to have a vascular problem as the cause of his or her bleed, physicians must decide whether to intervene, and if so, by what means (intraarterially, surgically, or both). For example, interventional radiologists can thread a thin wire through an artery in the leg, up to an AVM in the brain. Through an opening in the wire, a glue-like substance can be released, which will block the artery that supplies the malformation, eventually leading to obliteration of the malformation. In other cases, a neurosurgeon will cut out the malformation – tying off the blood vessels that lead to and away from it. Aneurysms can be treated by either approach, depending on the location and speed with which a solution is needed. Frequent brain imaging is required after these procedures, to make sure the problem has not recurred. If you have been diagnosed with one of these conditions, place an 'X' next to the goal of 'Repeat Brain Imaging.'

Amyloidosis:

Amyloidosis is a process of protein deposition in arteries. The effect is to weaken the arteries, allowing them to bleed more easily. An intracerebral hemorrhage in certain locations (lobar hemorrhages) makes one more suspicious of this diagnosis, especially if more than one occurs. It is also associated with the development of gradually worsening memory and cognitive (thinking) problems. If an elderly patient with memory problems experiences one or more non-traumatic lobar hemorrhages, this diagnosis is highly likely. Given that there is no treatment for amyloidosis, and that brain biopsy is required for the diagnosis, it is rarely proven during a person's lifetime.

Prevention: Unfortunately, there is not yet a cure for amyloidosis. General advice includes avoiding blood thinners, stimulants, smoking, and alcohol.

Tumors:

A benign or malignant tumor can be the source of bleeding in the brain. Many neurologists will perform an initial brain MRI/MRA at the time of a hemorrhagic stroke and then repeat the MRI/MRA in 3-4 months to check for an underlying tumor (after the blood has had time to clear).

Prevention: Tumors require the expertise of a neurologist or neurosurgeon to manage, and may also require an oncologist and radiation oncologist. The approach taken will depend on whether the tumor is benign, malignant, or a metastasis from another location in the body. If surgery or some other intervention has already occurred, place an 'X' next to the goal of 'Repeat Brain Imaging' on your Goal Chart.

Chapter 4: Putting It All Together

At this point, you will have read through Chapter 1 and, depending on your stroke type, either Chapter 2 or 3. You should also have placed an 'X' next to those goals on the Goal Chart that are appropriate for you. Most people will have many goals, while other may have only a few. You may also have needed to speak with your doctor about special circumstances or to get his or her input as to whether or not you suffer from atherosclerosis.

Now you can make the Goal Chart work for you. I recommend that you make a few photocopies of either the Ischemic or Hemorrhagic Goal Chart, whichever is appropriate for you, so that you can work with them. Your chart is a way to keep both yourself and your doctor organized as you reduce your stroke risk. Let's say that one of your goals is to lower your blood pressure to 120/80 or below. Each time you visit your doctor, you should write the date of your visit over the next available blank column to the right on the chart. When your blood pressure is taken in your doctor's office, either you or someone in the office should write that day's blood pressure under the column in the 'blood pressure at or below 120/80' row. If another of your goals is to have your LDL below 100 mg/dL, you will need to have your doctor send you for this blood test. Later, when you get the result, you can write it under that day's office date in the 'LDL less than 100 mg/dL' row. See the sample Goal Chart below:

"X"	GOAL NAME	SPECIFIC GOAL	Date 10-8-05	Date 1-13-06
	Blood Sugar	Control blood sugar so that HgA1c is less than 6.0		
X	Blood Pressure	Blood pressure at or below 120/80 mmHg (Consider thiazide diuretic or ACE inhibitor)	180/90	170/80
	No Smoking	Reduce and eventually stop smoking		
X	LDL	LDL less than 100 mg/dL	150	110

Clearly some goals are more difficult to achieve than others. For example, controlling your cholesterol with statin medications is usually much easier than losing weight or quitting smoking. The more difficult goals tend to be the ones that involve sustained discomfort and a permanent change in your habits. These goals are much more within your own control than your doctor's. On the other hand, since they are shared goals, your doctor may be able to help you by suggesting weight management programs, or providing you with diet and exercise advice. He or she may recommend classes for smoking cessation, or medications that can help you to quit smoking. Your doctor may even want to recommend another physician who is a specialist in treating your problem.

Once your goals are clearly before you, you will be surprised at how many ideas will occur to you as to how to achieve them. Just *having* clear goals helps you organize yourself in order to tackle them. You should try to see your doctor about once a month as the two of you work on these shared goals. You likely will feel a sense of achievement and control over your life as you complete them. Once you have completed them all, you will have done 99% of what can be done to prevent yourself from having a stroke, and should have a sense of satisfaction from doing what you can to prevent further strokes in your life.

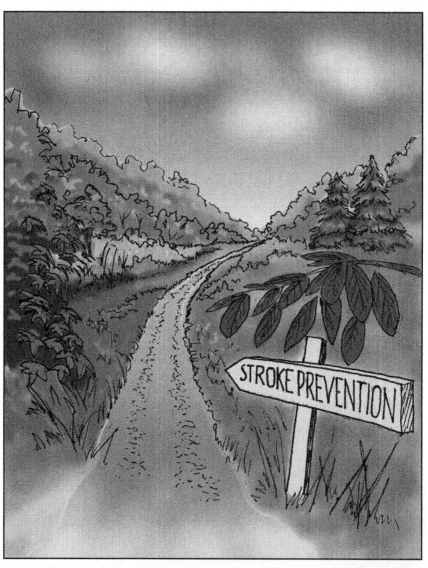

"Just *having* clear goals helps you organize yourself in order to tackle them."

Appendix A

Warfarin Use

Warfarin (brand name Coumadin) works by interfering with special proteins involved in blood clotting. The more warfarin you ingest, the 'thinner' (or less clot prone) your blood becomes. Warfarin requires much care to avoid under treatment or over treatment. Treatment effects are usually followed using the 'INR' (international normalization ratio), which measures the thinness of your blood. The usual goal INR is between 2.0-3.0. The higher the number, the less likely blood is to clot, but the more likely you are to bleed uncontrollably. If you have had trouble keeping your INR in the goal range, consider the following points:

(1) <u>Take warfarin consistently</u>: You must take your warfarin exactly as directed. Any missed doses, or extra doses, can dramatically change your INR.

(2) <u>Monitor your INR</u>: Monitor your INR at least once a month. It should be done more frequently if you are making dose changes or if your INR is not within the goal range.

(3) <u>Pay attention to vitamin K</u>: You must avoid taking supplemental vitamin K as well as be aware of which foods are rich in vitamin K (generally, green leafy vegetables, such as spinach or lettuce). You should either avoid these foods altogether, or attempt to eat them in a consistent manner, to avoid fluctuations in your INR.

(4) <u>Use brand Coumadin</u>: You may need to use brand name Coumadin (not the generic warfarin). Generic medications can vary in dosage from 80% to 125% of the brand dosage. Taking the brand name will eliminate this variability.

(5) <u>Be aware of medication interactions</u>: Before starting a new medication (especially antibiotics) or changing the dosage of an old medication, ask your doctor about potential interactions with warfarin. Either avoid the change or have your INR tested frequently to monitor the effect.

(6) <u>Consider home testing</u>: Consider obtaining a home testing machine if you require frequent INR testing and it is difficult for you to get to a blood drawing location.

Appendix B

What To Do If You're Having A Stroke

Although most people can significantly reduce their chances of having another stroke by following the advice in the preceding chapters, the risk unfortunately cannot be eliminated. Because of this concern, especially since you have already had a stroke or TIA, you should know what to do if you again experience symptoms suggestive of a stroke.

Those of you who have experienced an ischemic stroke or TIA probably experienced some combination of weakness on one side of the body, numbness, visual changes, difficulty walking, difficulty speaking and understanding, double-vision, or dizziness. Those of you who have experienced a hemorrhagic stroke may have experienced these same symptoms, along with a headache and perhaps confusion, sleepiness, or unconsciousness.

If you re-experience symptoms that are suggestive of a stroke, and are with someone at the time you experience these symptoms, have that person dial 911 and indicate to the operator the symptoms you are experiencing and that you might be having a stroke. If you cannot communicate with the people around you, you could dial 911 yourself and hand the phone to a person who is with you. If you are alone you should dial 911 yourself. Even if you are not able to communicate, the operators will be able to send the police or ambulance to your location, if you keep the phone off the hook. Also either you, or someone with you, should note the time your symptoms began, since this can affect what therapies are available to you in the hospital.

If you live with someone, it is best to discuss these issues with them ahead of time so they will be prepared should a stroke occur, especially since you may not be able to communicate with them during a stroke. Your loved ones or associates should know to immediately dial 911 on your behalf if you suddenly become unconscious.

In the case of a stroke, the paramedics' main objective is to get you to an emergency room as soon as possible. They might be able to help you immediately, though, by providing you with oxygen, giving you IV fluids if your blood pressure is low, giving you glucose if your blood sugar is low, and making sure you are not having an abnormal heart rhythm.

Once you are in an emergency room, the physicians will examine you to determine if they believe you are having a stroke. If they believe this to be the case, they will usually order a rapid CT scan of your head. This scan will allow them to determine immediately whether or not you are experiencing a hemorrhagic or an ischemic stroke.

In the case of a hemorrhagic stroke, they will often try to keep your blood pressure from rising too rapidly, make sure your blood isn't too thin (especially for those taking antiplatelet medications or warfarin), and possibly administer medications which reduce your chances of continued bleeding. Depending on the size of the hemorrhage, they may also call a neurosurgeon to determine if surgery would be beneficial to reduce the pressure on the brain. In the case of a subarachnoid hemorrhage, they may want to have you undergo a cerebral angiogram (providing detailed pictures of the arteries in your brain) to be sure you do not have an aneurysm (an arterial out pouching that can bleed easily).

In the case of an ischemic stroke, physicians will assess the timing or your stroke and how severe it is. If your ischemic stroke is not felt to be too severe or too minor, you may be offered a medication (tissue plasminogen activator or TPA) which can be administered through an IV and which may help to break up the clot which is presumably causing the stroke. In order to offer this IV medication, it must be administered within 3 hours of the onset of your symptoms. Whether or not to offer TPA is a difficult decision, since many conditions rule out the use of the medication, and since there is an increased risk of bleeding (in the brain and elsewhere) when it is used. If your stroke occurred greater than three but less than six hours prior, you may be offered TPA through intraarterial means. In this method of providing TPA, a wire is threaded into a leg artery and up to the location of the stroke. TPA is then released at the site of the arterial clot.

If you experience an ischemic stroke, but are not eligible for TPA, you likely will be given either IV heparin (a blood thinning agent) or an antiplatelet medication (aspirin, Aggrenox, Plavix, Ticlid). Physicians will also make sure that you have enough oxygen, that your blood glucose is kept within the normal range, that any infections are treated, and that your blood pressure is within a desirable range. Extensive testing is usually performed to try to determine the cause off the stroke.

Ischemic Stroke Goal Chart

"X"	GOAL NAME	Text Page	SPECIFIC GOAL
	Antiplatelet	8	Take an antiplatelet medication daily (aspirin, Aggrenox, Plavix, Ticlid)
	Blood Sugar	12	Control blood sugar so that HgA1c is less than 6.0
	Blood Pressure	14	Blood pressure at or below 120/80 mmHg (Consider thiazide diuretic or ACE inhibitor)
	No Smoking	15	Reduce and eventually stop smoking
	Alcohol	17	Less than or equal to 1 or 2 alcoholic drink(s) per day
	Aerobic Exercise	19	Aerobic exercise: 30 minutes at least three times per week
	Waist-toHip Ratio (WHR)	20	Women: Less than or equal to 0.86 Men: Less than or equal to 0.93
	Obstructive Sleep Apnea	22	Wear CPAP or BiPAP at night, consider surgery
	Impaired Glucose Tolerance	23	Consider special diet, oral medications
	LDL	24	LDL less than 100 mg/dL
	TG	24	TG less than 150 mg/dL
	HDL	24	HDL greater than 40 mg/dL
	Statin	25	Take a statin medication daily
	Homocysteine	26	Total Homocysteine less than 8 mmol/L
	Monitor INR	28	INR Goal _____
	Carotid Imaging	34	Periodic re-imaging should be performed (see text)

GOAL NAME	Date	Date	Date	Date	Date	Date
Antiplatelet						
Blood Sugar						
Blood Pressure						
No Smoking						
Alcohol						
Aerobic Exercise						
Waist-toHip Ratio (WHR)						
Obstructive Sleep Apnea						
Impaired Glucose Tolerance						
LDL						
TG						
HDL						
Statin						
Homocysteine						
Monitor INR						
Carotid Imaging						

Hemorrhagic Stroke Goal Chart

"X"	GOAL NAME	Text Page	SPECIFIC GOAL
	Repeat Brain Imaging	45 54 56	Preferably brain MRI with contast and MRA of head vessels
X	Blood Pressure	47	Blood pressure at or below 120/80 mmHg
	Alcohol	48	Avoid completely
	No Smoking	48	Reduce then stop smoking
	No Stimulants	50	Avoid: cocaine, amphetamines, dextroamphetamine, pemoline, methylphenidate, appetite suppressants, pseudoephedrine, phenylpropanolamine
	No Blood Thinners (unless advised by your doctor)	51	Avoid: aspirin, ibuprofen, Aggrenox, Plavix, Ticlid, Coumadin (warfarin)
	Monitor INR (If advised by your doctor)	51	INR Goal _____

72

GOAL NAME	Date	Date	Date	Date	Date	Date
Repeat Brain Imaging						
Blood Pressure						
Alcohol						
No Smoking						
No Stimulants						
No Blood Thinners (unless advised by your doctor)						
Monitor INR (If advised by your doctor)						

ENDNOTES

[1] MacMahon S, Peto R, Cutler J, Collins R, Sorlie P, Neaton J, Abbott R, Godwin J, Dyer A, Stamler J. *Lancet* 1990;335:765-774.

[2] Neal B, MacMahon S. *J Hypertension* 1995;13:1869-1873.

[3] Seventh Report of the Joint National Committee on the Prevention, Detection, Evaluation and Treatment of High Blood Pressure. *Hypertension.* 2004 Jan;43(1):1-3.

[4] Yusuf S, Sleight P, Pogue J, Bosch J, Davies R, Dagenais G. *New Engand Journal of Medicine* 2000 Jan 20;342(3):145-53

[5] Cushman WC. American Journal of Hypertension. 2003 Nov;16(11 Pt 2):31S-35S.

[6] ALLHAT Officers and Coordinators for the ALLHAT Collaborative Research Group. *Journal of the American Medical Association* 2002 288(23):2981-97.

[7] Shinton R, Beevers G. *British Medical Journal* 1989;298-94.

[8] Sacco RL, Roberts JK, Boden-Albala B, Gu Q, Lin IF, Kargman DE, Berglund L, Hauser WA, Shea S, Paik MC. *Stroke* 1997 May;28(5):929-35.

[9] Wolf PA, Belanger AJ, D'Agostino RB. *Neurologic clinics* 1992;10:177-91.

[10] Gill JS, Zezulka AV, Shipley MJ, Gill SK, Beevers DG. *New England Journal of Medicine.* 1986 Oct 23;315(17):1041-6.

[11] Camargo CA jr., *Stroke* 1989;20:1611-26.

[12] Sacco RL, Elkind ME, Boden-Albala B. The protective effect of moderate alcohol consumption on ischemic stroke, *Journal of the American Medical Association.* 1999;281:53-60.

[13] Berger K, Ajani UA, Kase CS, Gaziano JM, Buring JE, Glynn RJ, Hennekens CH. *New England Journal of Medicine.* 1999;341(21):1557-64.

[14] Kiely DK, Wolf PA, Cupples LA, Beiser AS, Kannel WB. *American Journal of Epidemiology* 1994;140(7):608-20.

[15] Sacco RL, Gan R, Boden-Albala B, Lin IF, Kargman DE, Hauser WA, Shea S, Paik MC. *Stroke* 1998;29(2):380-387.

[16] NIH Consensus Development Panel on Physical Activity and Cardiovascular health. Physical activity and cardiovascular

health. *Journal of the American Medical Association* 1996;276:241-6.

[17] Lean, M.E. Drugs Today. 2000 Nov;36(11):773-84.

[18] Rexrode KM, Hennekens CH, Willett WC, Colditz GA, Stampfer MJ, Rich-Edwards JW, Speizer FE, Manson JE.. *Journal of the American Medical Assocation* 1997 May 21;277(19):1539-45

[19] Lean, M.E. *Drugs Today* 2000 Nov;36(11):773-84.

[20] Suk SH, Sacco RL, Boden-Albala B, Cheun JF, Pittman JG, Elkind MS, Paik MC *Stroke* 2003 Jul;34(7):1586-92

[21] Qureshi A, Ballard RD *Journal of Allergy and Clinical Immunology* 2003 Oct;112(4):643-51; quiz 652.

[22] Kannel WB. *Journal of Atherosclerosis and Thrombosis* 2000; 6(2):60-6.

[23] Sacco RL, Benson RT, Kargman DE, Boden-Albala B, Tuck C, Lin IF, Cheng JF, Paik MC, Shea S, Berglund L. *Journal of the American Medical Assocation* 2001 Jun 6;285(21):2729-35.

[24] Amarenco P, Lavallee P, Touboul PJ. *Cerebrovascular Diseases* 2004;17 Suppl 1:81-8.

[25] Toole JF, Malinow MR, Chambless LE, Spence JD, Pettigrew LC, Howard VJ, Sides EG, Wang CH, Stampfer M. *Journal of the American Medical Assocation* 2004 Feb 4;291(5):565-75.

[26] Anderson CS, Feigin V, Bennett D, Lin RB, Hankey G, Jamrozik K; Australasian Cooperative Research on Subarachnoid Hemorrhage Study (ACROSS) Group. *Stroke* 2004 Mar;35(3):633-7.

[27] Ohkuma H, Tabata H, Suzuki S, Islam MS. *Stroke* 2003 Jan;34(1):96-100

[28] Isaksen J, Egge A, Waterloo K, Romner B, Ingebrigtsen T. *Journal of Neurology, Neurosurgery, and Psychiatry* 2002 Aug;73(2):185-7

[29] Kissela BM, Sauerbeck L, Woo D, Khoury J, Carrozzella J, Pancioli A, Jauch E, Moomaw CJ, Shukla R, Gebel J, Fontaine R, Broderick J. *Stroke* 2002 May;33(5):1321-6.

[30] Donahue RP, Abbott RD, Reed DM, Yano K. *Journal of the American Medical Assocation* 1986;255:2311-14.

[31] Stampfer MJ, Colditz GA, Willett WC, Speizer FE, Hennekens CH. *New England Journal of Medicine* 1988 Aug 4;319(5):267-73.

[32] Kissela BM, Sauerbeck L, Woo D, Khoury J, Carrozzella J, Pancioli A, Jauch E, Moomaw CJ, Shukla R, Gebel J, Fontaine R, Broderick J. *Stroke* 2002 May;33(5):1321-6.

[33] Kurth T, Kase CS, Berger K, Gaziano JM, Cook NR, Buring JE. *Stroke* 2003 Dec;34(12):2792-5

[34] Kurth T, Kase CS, Berger K, Schaeffner ES, Buring JE, Gaziano JM *Stroke* 2003 May;34(5):1151-5

[35] Thrift AG, McNeil JJ, Donnan GA. *Cerebrovascular Diseases* 1999 Jan-Feb;9(1):34-9.

[36] Wolf PA, Belanger AJ, D'Agostino RB. *Neurologic clinics* 1992;10:177-91.

About The Author

Dr. Alway is a board certified neurologist involved in stroke clinical trials research and full time private practice in Alexandria, Virginia. He is also the Chairman of the Stroke Clinical Effectiveness Team at Inova Alexandria Hospital. He regularly lectures physicians, physician's assistant students, and nurses regarding stroke treatment and prevention. In recognition of his teaching ability, he was elected to the national Alpha Omega Alpha honor society. You can visit his website, Stroke Doc (http://Strokedoc.typepad.com), to review recent news regarding stroke treatments and prevention. The website for his medical practice is: http://www.neuro-headache.com.